Bronchitis

Lung Disease

Management And Care Tips

By **CYNTHIA LEONARD**

TABLE OF CONTENTS

PART 1: Understanding Bronchitis

Introduction to Bronchitis

The respiratory ailment known as bronchitis is characterised by inflammation of the bronchial tubes - the airways that provide air to the lungs.

Increased mucus production, airway constriction and a variety of symptoms including coughing, breathing difficulties and chest pain are all caused by inflammation. **Acute** and **Chronic** bronchitis are the two primary forms of the illness.

Acute Bronchitis:

Cause: Viral infections, such as the flu or common cold viruses are often the cause of acute bronchitis. Bacterial infections may also sometimes be the cause.

Symptoms: A persistent cough that often produces mucus, weariness, chest pain and sometimes a low-grade fever are common symptoms.

Duration: With rest and supportive treatment, most cases of acute bronchitis cure on their own in a few weeks.

Chronic Bronchitis:

Cause: As chronic bronchitis is a more persistent ailment, it is often linked to smoking cigarettes or prolonged exposure to lung irritants like chemicals and dust from the workplace or air pollution.

Symptoms: Recurrent bouts of coughing and dyspnea are common in chronic bronchitis, in addition to a persistent cough and increased mucus production. The airways may sustain irreversible damage over time.

Duration: A kind of chronic obstructive lung disease, chronic bronchitis is a chronic illness that may linger for months or years *(COPD)*.

Common Bronchitis Symptoms

- ➤ Cough *(which may discharge mucus that is clear, yellow, green or even blood-tinged)*
- ➤ Breathlessness
- ➤ Pain or discomfort in the chest

> Weary
> Chills and a low temperature, *which are more typical with acute bronchitis*

Acute bronchitis often causes Sore throats.

TREATMENT

Supportive care is usually the primary course of therapy for acute bronchitis. This includes getting enough sleep, drinking enough of water, using expectorants or cough suppressants as required and controlling symptoms.

Chronic Bronchitis: Reducing smoking, avoiding allergens in the air and utilising bronchodilators or inhaled corticosteroids to increase airflow are all common lifestyle modifications that are used to manage chronic bronchitis.

For an accurate diagnosis and suitable therapy, it is important to speak with a healthcare provider, particularly in cases when symptoms are severe, chronic or there is a history of respiratory disorders.

PART 2: Diagnosis and Medical Insights

Seeking Professional Help

The following actions may be taken to get medical attention for bronchitis:

Making an appointment with your primary care provider is advised. They may assess your medical history, go over your symptoms and provide a physical examination.

Walk-in Clinic or Urgent Care: If you are unable to see your primary care physician right away, you may want to visit a walk-in clinic or an urgent care facility. They are able to provide prompt treatment and assessment.

Telehealth Services: You may have a remote consultation with a medical expert thanks to the telehealth services provided by some healthcare providers. If you are unable to attend a physical site, this might be quite helpful.

Emergency Room: Get emergency medical assistance right away if you have severe symptoms including breathing difficulties, ongoing chest discomfort, disorientation or pale lips or face.

Consultation with a Specialist: If you need more testing and care, your primary care physician may refer you to a pulmonologist or respiratory specialist.

Be ready to discuss your symptoms, their length, any pertinent medical history and any prescription or over-the-counter drugs you are taking with a healthcare provider. The medical professional will be better able to diagnose patients and suggest the best course of action with the use of this information.

It is essential to treat chronic respiratory symptoms since they may indicate bacterial or viral infections that need to be treated specifically, leading to bronchitis. You may avoid problems and properly manage your symptoms with the guidance of a medical professional.

Diagnostic Tests for Bronchitis

The goals of bronchitis diagnostic testing are to evaluate the severity of symptoms, rule out other explanations and choose the best course of action for therapy. The following are some typical bronchitis diagnosis tests:

Physical Assessment:
In addition to reviewing your medical history, the doctor will examine you physically and use a stethoscope to listen to your lungs.

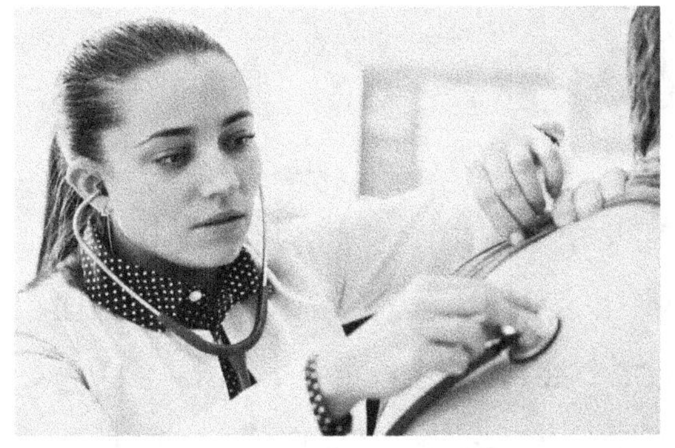

Inquiries about symptoms including cough, dyspnea and chest pain may also be made.

Chest X-ray:
To rule out pneumonia or other respiratory disorders, a chest X-ray may be prescribed. It may assist the

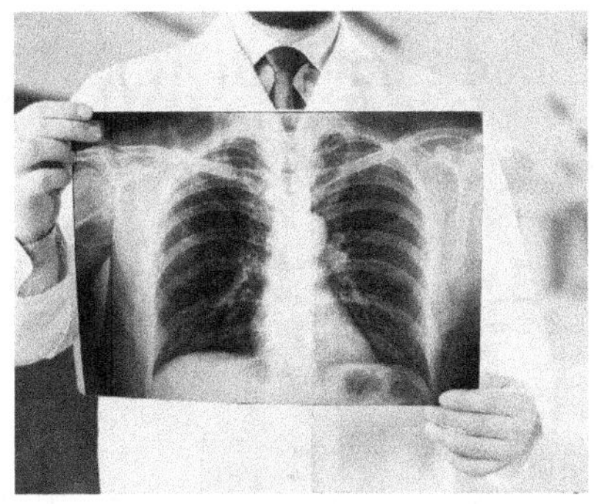

physician in seeing the lungs and determining any anomalies.

Tests for Pulmonary function (PFTs):

These examinations gauge how effectively your lungs are working. One popular PFT for evaluating lung function and airflow is spirometry. It might assist in figuring out if the airways are restricted or obstructed.

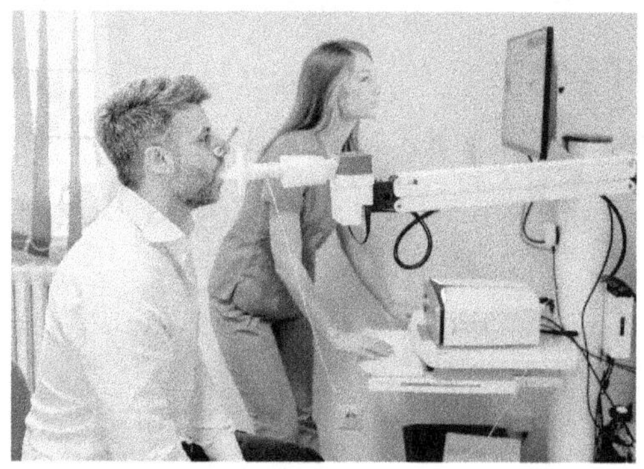

Sputum Culture:

Sputum or mucus coughed up from the lungs, may be collected and submitted to a laboratory for sensitivity testing and culture if the bronchitis is thought to be bacterial in origin. This may assist in figuring out which particular bacteria are causing the illness and which drug works best.

Blood Examinations:

To evaluate the patient's general health and rule out other possible causes of symptoms, blood tests may be performed.

Test for Arterial Blood Gas (ABG): By measuring the blood's concentrations of carbon dioxide and oxygen, this test may tell us how effectively our lungs are exchanging gases.

CT Scan:

To provide more precise pictures of the lungs and associated 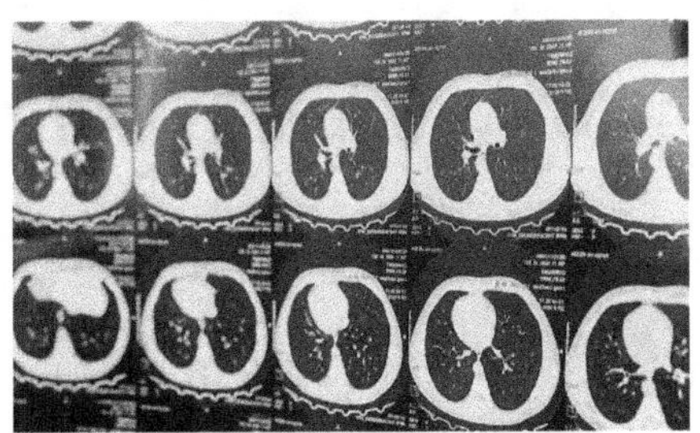 tissues, a computed tomography *(CT)* scan of the chest may be prescribed in certain circumstances.

Note that the precise tests carried out might change depending on the particular situation and the intensity of symptoms. While chronic bronchitis may need more involved testing to evaluate lung function and rule out other illnesses, acute bronchitis is often diagnosed simply on clinical symptoms and a physical examination.

Understanding Treatment Options

The underlying cause and kind of bronchitis determine the available treatment choices. *Here are a few broad recommendations:*

1. Rest and Drinking Water: Severe Bronchitis In order for the body to combat the illness, rest is essential. Maintaining hydration makes mucus less thick and easier to remove.

2. Medication: Infection of the Bronchi:

3. Analgesics and fever reducers: Acetaminophen and ibuprofen, two over-the-counter pain medications, may aid with symptoms.

4. Cough suppressants: In some situations, they may be used to treat a chronic cough.

5. Bronchodilators: To open airways, bronchodilators may be administered if wheezing is a symptom of bronchitis.

For Prolonged Bronchitis

6. Bronchodilators: These medications facilitate breathing by widening the airways.
7. Steroids: To lessen airway inflammation, a doctor may give inhaled corticosteroids.

8. Mucolytics: Drugs known as **"mucolytics"** thin mucus, which facilitates coughing.

9. Drugs known as antibiotics:

Antibiotics are often not administered for acute bronchitis unless a bacterial infection is present, since the majority of cases are viral.

In the event that a bacterial infection is causing the symptoms of chronic bronchitis, prescription antibiotics may be necessary.

10. DIY Solutions:
- **Humidifiers:** Increasing the moisture content of the air helps relieve congested respiratory tracts.
- Inhaling steam may also aid in the loosening of mucus.
- Gargling with warm saltwater might help relieve sore throats.

11. Modifications to Lifestyle:
Quitting smoking is crucial to preventing additional damage to the airways in cases of chronic bronchitis.

Steer Clear of Irritants: Reduce your exposure to allergens and contaminants in the environment.

12. Confirmation:
For the purpose of monitoring and treating chronic bronchitis in particular, routine examinations may be required.

For the correct diagnosis and course of treatment, always seek the advice of a healthcare provider.

As soon as symptoms develop or continue, get medical help. Also, treatment strategies may need to take certain factors into account for those with impaired immune systems or pre-existing medical disorders.

Medications and Their Role

Drugs can treat the symptoms of bronchitis and in some situations, its underlying causes. It's important to remember that antibiotics should only be used in situations of bacterial infection and are often ineffective for viral bronchitis.

Bronchodilators:

Albuterol and other **short-acting** bronchodilators are examples of drugs that help relax the muscles around the airways, facilitating easier breathing. They are often used to treat acute bronchitis in order to reduce symptoms like wheezing and dyspnea.

When treating chronic bronchitis, **long-acting** bronchodilators *(such as salmeterol and formoterol)* are usually utilised to increase airflow and give long-lasting relief. They often feature in the regimen for those with COPD or chronic obstructive lung disease.

Corticosteroids:

Inhaled corticosteroids: Drugs like budesonide and fluticasone, for example, may help lessen airway inflammation. They are often used to control symptoms and stop exacerbations of COPD and chronic bronchitis.

Oral corticosteroids, such as prednisone: To rapidly decrease inflammation and improve breathing, a brief course of oral corticosteroids may be recommended in severe instances or exacerbations of chronic bronchitis.

Mucolytic agents:

N-acetylcysteine (NAC): This drug thins and loosens mucus, facilitating its removal from the respiratory system. It may help with the symptoms of chronic bronchitis and lessen how often exacerbations occur.

Antibiotics:

If a bacterial infection is present: Antibiotics *(such as azithromycin and amoxicillin)* may be recommended if there is a possibility that the cause of the acute bronchitis is a bacterial infection.

Antibiotics work against viral infections, therefore it's critical to identify if the illness is bacterial before taking any medication.

Relieversers of Pain and Fever:

Acetaminophen or ibuprofen: These over-the-counter drugs may help lower fever and ease bronchitis-related discomfort.

PART 3: Lifestyle Changes for Better Lung Health

Importance of Quitting Smoking

Given its many positive effects on one's health, relationships and finances, quitting smoking is crucial for a number of reasons. *The following are some major arguments emphasising how crucial it is to stop smoking:*

Advantages for Health:

Lower Risk of Diseases: Smoking is a major risk factor for a number of dangerous illnesses, such as heart disease, lung cancer, stroke and respiratory problems including chronic obstructive pulmonary disease (COPD).

Reducing smoking substantially lowers the chance of developing these illnesses.

Better Respiratory Health: Giving up smoking improves lung function and lowers the risk of respiratory infections and illnesses including pneumonia and bronchitis.

Improved Cardiovascular Health: Smoking raises the risk of heart disease and stroke by damaging the cardiovascular system. Giving up smoking lowers the risk of certain cardiovascular problems and improves blood circulation.

Extended Life Expectancy

Extended Life Span: Research continuously demonstrates that stopping smoking prolongs life. It helps people live healthier and longer lives.

Enhanced Life Quality

Improved Physical Fitness: Smoking may harm one's ability to be physically fit and resilient. People who stop smoking may benefit from increased energy, endurance and general physical well-being.

Improved Mental Health: Anxiety and depression are two mental health conditions that are linked to smoking. Better mental and cognitive health may result from quitting smoking.

Savings in money

Cost Savings: Giving up smoking might save a lot of money since it's a costly habit. Spending money on cigarettes may go towards other important things, including leisure and health.

Social Advantages:

Decreased Social Stigma: People who stop smoking might escape the stigma attached to smoking as it becomes less socially acceptable. It also encourages a more salubrious social milieu.

Defending Others:

Secondhand Smoke: Giving up smoking has advantages for the smoker as well as for others as it shields people from secondhand smoke's damaging effects. This is especially essential for family members, friends and coworkers.

Child Health and Pregnancy:

Better Pregnancy Outcomes: Smoking during pregnancy has been connected to a number of problems, such as low birth weight and premature delivery. Giving up smoking is essential for the health of the mother and the foetus.

Diminished Effect on the Environment:

Environmental Conservation: The production and disposal of cigarettes damage the environment. Giving up smoking contributes to lessening the waste and manufacture of tobacco products' negative environmental effects.
Giving up smoking is mandatory for enhancing one's own health, extending one's life, saving money and creating a more positive and encouraging social atmosphere.

Benefits accrue not just to the person but also to those in their immediate vicinity. People may get help from a variety of support systems, such as community programmes, medicine, and counselling to help them stop smoking.

Nutrition and Diet Tips

Although there is no treatment for bronchitis, a healthy diet is essential for maintaining general health and promoting the body's natural healing processes.

These following food and nutrition advice will help you manage your bronchitis:

Maintain Hydration:

Water, herbal teas and broths are good sources of fluids that may help keep your respiratory tract wet and aid in the removal of mucus.

Include Foods That Reduce Inflammation:
Eat a diet high in anti-inflammatory foods to help lower respiratory system inflammation.
Fruits *(cherries, berries, citrus fruits)*, vegetables *(broccoli, tomatoes, leafy greens)*, and fatty fish *(salmon, mackerel)* are some examples.

Rich in Vitamin C Foods:

The immune system may be supported by vitamin C. Add bell peppers, broccoli, strawberries, kiwis and citrus fruits to your diet.

Foods High in Zinc:

Immune system performance depends on zinc. Add foods high in zinc, such as beans, nuts, shellfish, poultry and lean meats.

Consumption of Protein:

Sufficient protein is necessary for immune system support and tissue repair. Eat a diet rich in lean meats, poultry, fish, eggs, dairy, legumes and nuts.

Onions with Garlic:

Onions and garlic are both antibacterial and anti-inflammatory. Include them in your meals to boost your immunity even more. **The Fatty Acids Omega-3:**

Flaxseeds, chia seeds, walnuts and fatty fish are among the foods high in omega-3 fatty acids that may help lower inflammation and promote general health.

Steer clear of irritants:

Eat less or stay away from items that might irritate the respiratory system, such as meals that are spicy, dairy products *(if they increase mucus production)*, and foods that you could be sensitive to and cause allergies.

Warm and Comforting Beverages:

Warm liquids that soothe the throat, such as ginger tea, warm water with honey or herbal teas, may assist.

Little, Regular Meals:

Your respiratory system may handle smaller, more frequent meals better than bigger, heavier ones.

The Power of Regular Exercise

Frequent exercise may be quite helpful in boosting respiratory health in general and can be especially helpful for those who are coping with bronchitis.

Inflammation of the bronchial tubes, which transport air to and from the lungs, is a hallmark of bronchitis. The degree of symptoms may need modifications to an exercise regimen.

Some ways that consistent physical activity might help manage bronchitis:

Enhanced Respiratory Performance:

Frequent exercise improves respiratory muscle strength, which increases the muscles' ability to move air into and out of the lungs.

With time, lung capacity may be increased by aerobic sports like swimming, cycling or brisk walking, which will increase the effectiveness of oxygen exchange.

Boosted Immune Response:

An increase in immunity has been linked to regular physical exercise. An enhanced immune system is more effective in warding off infections, particularly those that could exacerbate bronchitis.

Clearance of Mucus:

Exercise may increase mucus production in the airways, which helps to eliminate germs and allergens. Those who suffer from bronchitis may find this very helpful as it may lessen congestion.

Mitigation of Respiratory Symptoms:

Moderate-intensity exercises may help control symptoms and enhance general well-being, while intense activity may make symptoms worse during acute periods of bronchitis.

Incorporating breathing exercises, such pursed lip breathing, into a fitness regimen helps improve the strength and control of the respiratory muscles.

Advantages for Cardiovascular Health:

Regular cardiovascular exercise enhances circulation and heart health. This may be quite important for those who have

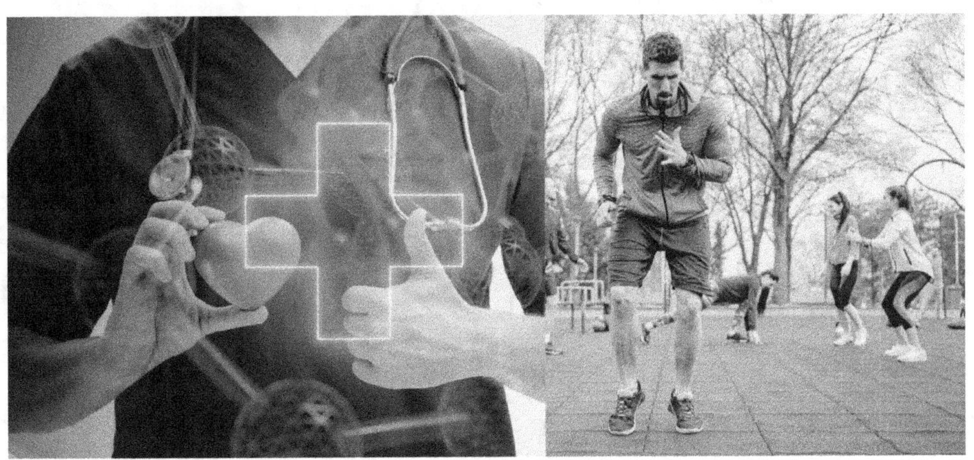

bronchitis because it makes sure that oxygen gets to all of the different tissues and organs in an effective manner.

Controlling Weight:

Regular exercise combined with a healthy weight helps lessen the strain on the respiratory system. Gaining too much weight may aggravate respiratory conditions and strain the lungs.

Psychological Advantages:

Bronchitis is one of the chronic respiratory diseases that may be psychologically exhausting. Exercise has been shown to lower stress, anxiety and sadness, which improves quality of life for those with bronchitis overall.

Note that people with bronchitis should always speak with their doctor before beginning or adjusting an exercise programme, particularly if the illness is severe.

Exercise must be managed with a customised strategy that takes into account each person's unique symptoms and health state in order to be both safe and successful in treating bronchitis.

Stress Management Techniques

Stress may impair immunity and increase susceptibility to infections, especially respiratory infections like bronchitis, even if it may not be the primary cause of bronchitis.

Stress may sometimes make symptoms worse and make healing more difficult. As a result, stress management is crucial for general health as well as for promoting bronchitis recovery.

The following stress-reduction methods might be useful:

Breathing Techniques:

To ease tension and encourage relaxation, try deep breathing techniques. Inhale via your nose and exhale through your mouth while you concentrate on taking calm, deep breaths.
Meditation with mindfulness:

Use mindfulness meditation as a way to focus on the here and now. This may lessen tension and anxiety. For newcomers, apps or other tools with guided meditation might be beneficial.

PMR, or Progressive Muscle Relaxation:

PMR entails tensing and releasing your body's various muscle groups. This method encourages relaxation and aids in the release of bodily stress.

Yoga:

Mild yoga may enhance general wellbeing and reduce stress. Select positions that you find comfortable and concentrate on slow, deliberate breathing and moderate stretching.

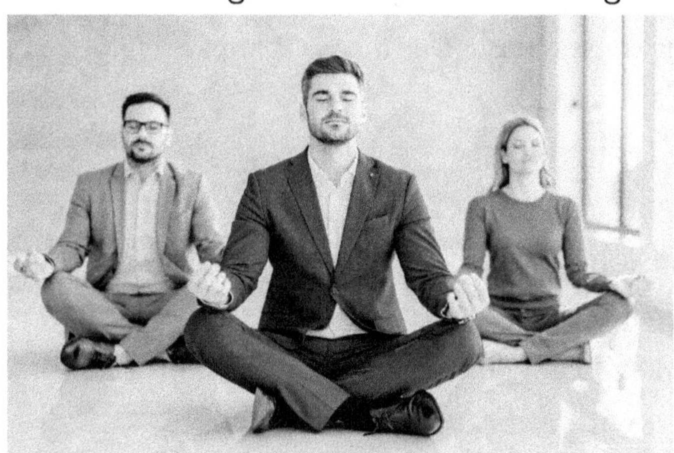

Warm Baths:

To calm your thoughts and relax your body, take warm showers. The relaxing effect might be strengthened by adding Epsom salts or essential oils like lavender.

Sufficient Sleep and Rest:

Make sure you have enough rest and sleep. Making sleep a priority is essential for healing since fatigue may exacerbate stress.

Choosing a Healthier Lifestyle:

Eat a healthy, balanced diet, drink enough water and abstain from stimulants like too much alcohol or coffee. These lifestyle decisions may enhance your general wellbeing.

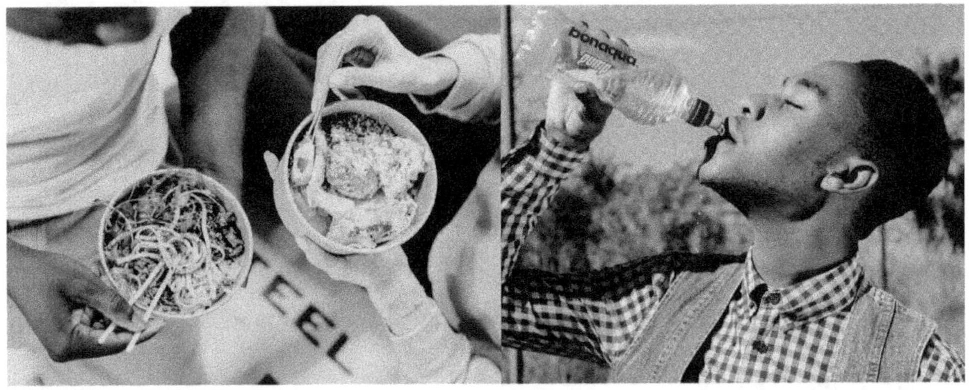

Writing with Expression:

Writing in a journal about your ideas and emotions may be a therapeutic method of stress relief. Write about your thoughts, feelings and experiences with bronchitis and other facets of life.

Social Assistance:

Make contact with loved ones, friends or support networks. Stress may be reduced and emotional support can be obtained by talking about your experiences and emotions.

Effective Time Management:

Plan out your daily tasks to lessen the stress that comes with time constraints. Set priorities for your projects and divide them into doable chunks.

Expert Assistance:

If stress becomes too much to handle, think about getting professional mental health assistance. They may provide direction and encouragement for efficient stress management.

PART 4: Home Remedies and Natural Approaches

Herbal Therapies

Although the effectiveness of herbal treatments for bronchitis is not well supported by research, several plants are thought to offer potential advantages for respiratory health.

It's important to remember that these therapies shouldn't be used in lieu of traditional medical care and that getting advice from a healthcare provider is necessary for an accurate diagnosis and course of treatment!

Furthermore, each person will react differently to herbal therapies and it's important to think about any possible drug interactions.

These plants are often believed to have respiratory benefits:

Eucalyptus:

When using steam inhalation to assist clear congestion and open the airways, eucalyptus oil is often employed.

It could be able to fight respiratory infections thanks to its antibacterial qualities.

Ginger:

Because of its anti-inflammatory and antioxidant qualities, ginger may help with symptoms including sore throats and coughs.

Honey blended with ginger or ginger tea may be calming.

Mint Pepper:

Menthol, which is found in peppermint, has the ability to assist breathing by relaxing the muscles in the respiratory system.

Breathing in vapours of peppermint oil or drinking peppermint tea might help.

Root Licorice:

Because licorice root is said to have anti-inflammatory qualities, it might help relieve throat discomfort.

It may be purchased as a tea, but extended usage is to be avoided because of possible negative consequences.

Thyme:

It is believed that thyme has antibacterial qualities, which might aid in treating respiratory infections.

Consider making thyme tea or using thyme in your food.

Oregano:

Antimicrobial substances found in oregano may help strengthen the immune system.

Although it is potent, oregano oil should be used with caution when using it.

Pure Honey:

Due to its calming properties for the throat, honey has been used for centuries.

You may drink it on its own or mix it with herbal drinks *(don't give honey to babies however)*.

Turmeric:
Due to its antioxidant and anti-inflammatory qualities, turmeric may help maintain respiratory health.
It could be advantageous to drink turmeric tea or add turmeric to food.

Certain herbs may trigger adverse responses or interact negatively with medicines. As soon as symptoms develop or continue, get medical help.

Breathing Exercises

For those who have bronchitis, breathing exercises may assist to enhance oxygenation, improve lung function and support general respiratory health. Please note that these exercises should be done slowly and if you have severe bronchitis or any other respiratory ailment, you should contact a healthcare practitioner before beginning any new exercise plan.

The following breathing techniques might be helpful for those who have bronchitis:

Pursed-Lip Inhalation:

- Take two calm breaths through your nose.
- As if you're about to whistle, purse your lips.
- Breathe out four times through pursed lips, slowly and softly.

By keeping the airways open for a longer period of time, pursed-lip breathing lessens breathing effort and enhances carbon dioxide and oxygen exchange.

Deep breathing or diaphragmatic breathing:

- Comfortably lay down or sit, grasp your belly with one hand and your chest with the other.

- Take a slow, deep breath through your nose, letting your belly fill up instead of your chest.

- Feel your belly drop as you gently release breath through pursed lips.

Deep, slow breaths are encouraged by diaphragmatic breathing, which also serves to develop the diaphragm, the primary breathing muscle.

Breathing in Segments:

- With your back straight, choose a comfortable seat.

- Put your hands on your abdomen and chest.

- Breathe in softly, filling one side of your lungs at a time.

- Fill the lower lungs first, followed by the middle and lastly the upper lungs.
- Slowly exhale in the other direction.

Increased ventilation and better lung expansion may be achieved by segmental breathing.

ACBT or the Active Cycle of Breathing Techniques:

Breathe in deeply through your nose and out slowly through pursed lips. This is controlled breathing.

Exercises for thoracic expansion:

Breathe in deeply, then out quickly to assist clear the airways of mucus.

Forced expiratory technique:

In order to expel mucus from the lungs, inhale deeply and cough.

Breathing exercises known as ACBT are often advised for those suffering from long-term respiratory disorders, such as bronchitis.

Always start out softly and work your way up to longer and more intense workouts depending on how comfortable you are.

Steam Inhalation Benefits

One popular at-home treatment for bronchitis and other respiratory ailments is steam inhalation. Although it may not be a cure for bronchitis, it might help reduce some of the pain that comes with the illness.

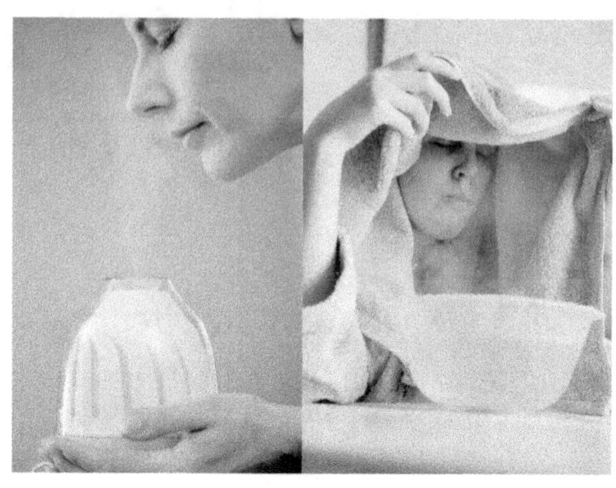

A few possible advantages of steam inhalation for bronchitis:

Moisturises Airways: Breathing in steam has the effect of moisturising and calming the airways, which is especially advantageous if you have bronchitis. The moisture in the air helps ease dryness and discomfort in the bronchial passages and throat.

Mucus Loosening: Inhaling steam may aid in the release of mucus and phlegm from the respiratory tract, facilitating its removal by coughing. This is particularly useful in cases of bronchitis, since increased mucus production is often seen as a symptom.

Reduces Congestion: Breathing becomes easier when clogged nasal passages and airways are opened up by the warmth and moisture of steam. This may be especially helpful if you have both bronchitis and nasal congestion.

Calms Irritation: Inflammation and irritation of the bronchial passages are common side effects of bronchitis. Steam inhalation may help relax these inflamed airways and provide momentary respite from symptoms such as wheezing and coughing.

Helps Expectoration: The body may eliminate mucus and allergens from the respiratory system via expectoration, which is aided by steam inhalation. This may facilitate better breathing and airway clearance.

This is how steam inhalation is done:

- Water is boiled in a pot.
- After taking the pot off of the hob, set it down on a level surface.
- *If desired,* add a few drops of essential oils, such as peppermint or eucalyptus **(optional)**.
- Lean over the pot while maintaining a safe distance to prevent burns, making a tent out of a towel over your head.

- Take short pauses if the steam becomes too hot or unpleasant as you inhale it for 5 to 10 minutes.

It's important to remember that while inhaling steam might help, it cannot replace medical care.

Creating a Respiratory-Friendly Environment

Establishing a space that is conducive to breathing is essential for those who are coping with bronchitis.

These advice may be used to assist someone with bronchitis breathe easier:

Dust-free and spotless surroundings:

To reduce airborne allergens, dust and clean your living areas on a regular basis.

To collect dust particles, use a moist cloth or a hoover cleaner equipped with a **HEPA** filter.

Add Humidity to the Air:

Keep the humidity at a suitable range (30–50%) to avoid the air being too dry, which might irritate the respiratory system. To add moisture to the air, use a cool-mist humidifier.

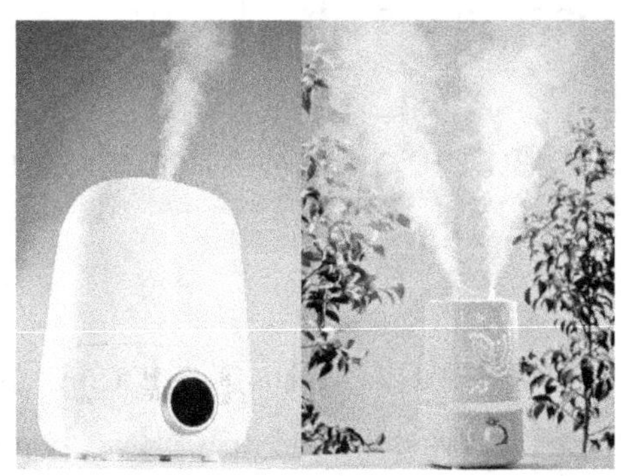

Airflow:

Make sure there's enough airflow by utilising fans or opening windows.

Steer clear of smoke, fumes and strong odours since they might exacerbate respiratory difficulties.

Steer clear of Allergens:

Recognise and reduce your exposure to allergens, including mould, pollen and pet dander.

Consider covering pillows and mattresses with allergen-proof materials.

Cleanse the Air:

To capture airborne particles, use air purifiers equipped with **HEPA** filters.

Think about putting indoor plants, such as spider or snake plants, that are believed to have air-purifying properties.

Maintain Hydration:

To assist release mucus and keep the respiratory tract wet, drink plenty of water.

Soups and teas that are heated may be calming and help you stay hydrated.

Warm Compresses:

Warm compresses should be applied to the chest to ease discomfort and reduce congestion.

Raising Your Sleeping Position:

To raise the upper body as you sleep, utilise pillows or an adjustable bed. This may facilitate better breathing and less coughing.

Steer clear of Irritants:

Avoid breathing in tobacco smoke and other allergens.

Select hypoallergenic or fragrance-free home items.

Maintain Appropriate Respiratory Hygiene:

Promote frequent hand washing to stop the transmission of illnesses.

When sneezing or coughing, cover your mouth and nose with tissues or elbows.

Stay Warm:

Wear warm clothing to protect yourself from the chilly air, which might cause bronchial spasms.

Observe Medical Advice

Follow **medical experts'** instructions about the use of prescribed drugs and treatment regimens.

Keep your follow-up visits and let your doctor know if your symptoms change.

PART 5: Practical Tips for Going About Your Daily Life.

Travelling with Bronchitis

Travelling with bronchitis can be challenging, as it can worsen symptoms and slow recovery.

To ensure a safe journey, consult with a healthcare professional before making travel plans. Follow medical advice, including prescription medications or specific precautions.

Stay hydrated by drinking plenty of fluids to keep your respiratory system moist. If your bronchitis is severe, postpone air travel due to dry air and changes in air pressure.

Pack all necessary medications, including antibiotics or bronchodilators and keep a copy of your prescription. Protect yourself from germs by practising good hygiene, such as frequent handwashing and avoiding contact with sick individuals.

Dress appropriately by dressing in layers and bringing a scarf to cover your mouth and nose in cold or dry environments. Plan for enough rest and relaxation, avoid overexertion and listen to your body.

Consider travel insurance that covers medical emergencies to provide peace of mind. Inform your travel companions about your condition and know how to respond in case of an emergency.

HANDLING SEASONAL DIFFICULTIES

It takes a mix of preventative steps, symptom management and seeking medical guidance when required to treat bronchitis during seasonal changes.

The following advice may assist manage seasonal bronchitis-related difficulties:

Rainy Season and Winter - Maintain Hydration:

Make sure you stay hydrated by consuming plenty of room temperature or warm water, herbal teas and clear broths.

Drinking enough water might help relieve sore throats and keep the airways moist.

Adjust the Humidity in Your Space:

To add moisture to the air, use a humidifier. This may lessen coughing and soothe respiratory tract inflammation. In order to stop germs and mould from growing, make sure you clean the humidifier on a regular basis.

In All Seasons - ***Avoid Health hazard irritants:***

Avoiding irritants such as smoking and strong odours might help relieve the symptoms of bronchitis.

This covers air fresheners, strong cleaning agents and secondhand smoking.

Maintain Proper Hand Hygiene:

To lessen the chance of bacterial and viral infections that might exacerbate bronchitis, wash your hands often.

To stop the transmission of germs, avoid touching your face, particularly your lips and nose.

Use a Nasal Rinse with Saline:

By removing mucus from the nasal passages, saline nasal rinses may ease congestion and facilitate better breathing.

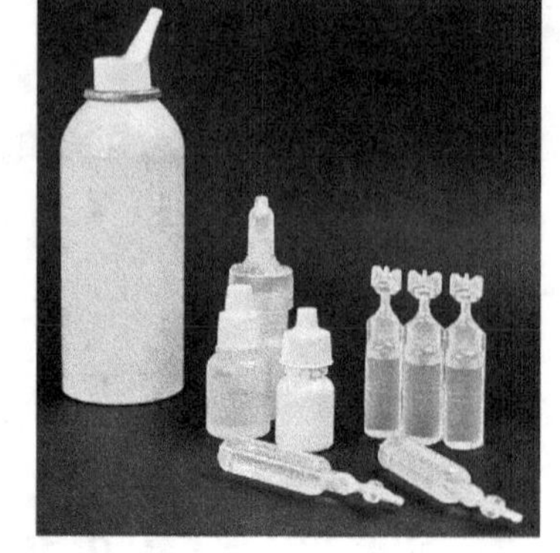

This is especially helpful if nasal congestion is present along with bronchitis.

Relaxation & Rest:

Make sure you get enough sleep so your body can recover. Steer clear of activities that put a load on your breathing system.

Make Use of Warm Compress:

To ease pain in your chest and encourage relaxation, place a warm compress on your back or chest.

Over-the-Counter Drugs:

Expectorants and cough suppressants available over-the-counter may help relieve congestion and coughing.

Always take medication as prescribed and see a doctor if your symptoms don't go away or if you have any concerns.

Breathe in the Steam:

One way to reduce congestion and release mucus is to inhale steam.

This may be achieved by breathing in steam from a bowl of hot water or by having a hot shower.

Speak with a Medical Professional:

Seek medical help if your symptoms become worse or stay the same. They are able to rule out any difficulties, provide an accurate diagnosis and suggest suitable treatments.

This is only general advice and may not work for everyone. It's important to speak with a doctor / medical expert for tailored guidance on your particular circumstances.

Balancing Work and Health

During bronchitis recovery, it is mandatory to balance work and health to ensure a smooth and efficient recovery.

To do this, prioritise rest, communicate with your employer, set realistic work expectations, take sick leave if necessary, create a flexible work schedule, maintain a balanced diet, practise good hygiene, use breathing techniques and incorporate light physical activity.

Please know that everyone's recovery process is different, so listen to your body and make adjustments as needed.

A balanced diet and proper hydration are crucial for your smooth recovery and consuming nutritious foods and staying well-hydrated can support your immune system.

Regular hand washing, using hand sanitizer and avoiding close contact with colleagues can help prevent the spread of the illness.

Use deep breathing exercises to open up airways and promote healing, especially during work breaks or moments of stress.

Gentle activities like short walks or stretching can improve circulation and lung function. Consult with your doctor to ensure you are following the right treatment plan and any additional precautions.

Prioritising your health during bronchitis recovery will lead to a quicker and more successful return to your regular work routine. By following these tips, you can ensure a smooth and efficient recovery process while fulfilling your professional responsibilities.

PART 6: Supportive Alternative Approaches

Pulmonary Rehabilitation

For those with long-term respiratory disorders, such as bronchitis, **Pulmonary rehabilitation** may be an important part of the healing process.

A comprehensive programme called pulmonary rehabilitation is meant to enhance the general health and functional capacity of those suffering from long-term respiratory conditions. Although it is often advised for ailments such as chronic obstructive pulmonary disease *(COPD)*, those recuperating from bronchitis may also find it beneficial.

The following are some essential elements of pulmonary rehabilitation for the recuperation of bronchitis:

Education: To assist patients better comprehend their illness, pulmonary rehabilitation programmes often incorporate educational components. This might include being knowledgeable about the causes, signs and efficient treatment options of bronchitis.

Breathing Exercises: To enhance lung function and efficiency, respiratory therapists often lead patients through a variety of breathing exercises. These exercises have the potential to improve total respiratory muscle strength and lessen dyspnea.

Physical Exercise: A key component of pulmonary rehabilitation is the implementation of structured exercise programmes. These activities, which might include strength training, flexibility training and cardiovascular exercises are customised to each person's ability.

Frequent exercise improves general health, endurance and cardiovascular fitness.

Nutritional Advice: Eating a balanced diet is important for good health in general and for respiratory health in particular.

Programmes for pulmonary rehabilitation may include dietary advice to support people in making educated food choices.

Psychosocial assistance: It may be difficult to manage a chronic respiratory illness, therefore it's important to have psychosocial assistance. Programmes for pulmonary rehabilitation may include therapy or support groups to treat the psychological and emotional components of having bronchitis.

Medication Management: Participants may get instruction on how to take drugs correctly, including how to utilise inhalers and how to take prescriptions as directed.

NOTE that the precise elements of pulmonary rehabilitation might change based on the requirements of the patient as well as the programme. It is recommended to speak with medical specialists who can evaluate the patient's condition and provide a suitable rehabilitation plan if you or someone you know is recovering from bronchitis and considering pulmonary rehabilitation.

Acupuncture and Bronchitis

In order to enhance energy flow **(Qi)** and aid in healing, acupuncture is a traditional Chinese medical procedure that includes inserting tiny needles into certain body locations.

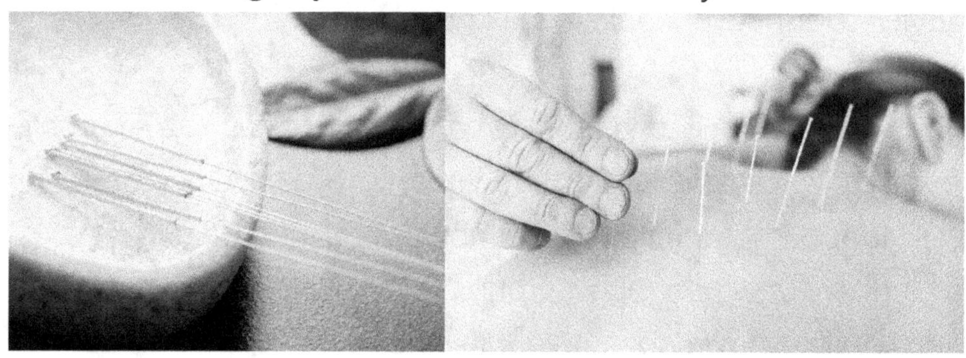

Although acupuncture is often used to treat a variety of illnesses, its efficacy for treating some illnesses, such as bronchitis, is still being investigated and debated.

Viral infections are often the cause of acute bronchitis, although long-term exposure to irritants like smoking is frequently linked to chronic bronchitis.

When it comes to treating bronchitis, acupuncture as a stand-alone therapy has little scientific backing.

Nonetheless, a few studies indicate that acupuncture could be useful in treating symptoms including inflammation, dyspnea and coughing.

Acupuncture for bronchitis may be considered in the following ways:

Symptom Relief: Breathing difficulties and coughing are two common bronchitis symptoms that acupuncture may assist with. It is believed to do this via encouraging calmness and lowering inflammation.

Immune System Support: Some people think that acupuncture might boost immunity, which could help the body fight off infections, particularly bronchitis-causing ones.

Energy Balance: Qi, or energy, in the body is seen as the foundation of health in traditional Chinese medicine. The goal of acupuncture is to reestablish equilibrium and supporters claim that this may have a favourable effect on a number of illnesses, including respiratory problems.

Although some people claim success with acupuncture, outcomes might differ and more study is required to determine whether or not it is particularly effective for bronchitis. **It is not appropriate** to replace traditional medical treatments with acupuncture, particularly in instances that are severe or persistent.

Speak with a licensed healthcare provider if you are thinking about trying acupuncture for bronchitis or any other illness. They can provide advice specific to your requirements and situation and can assist you in making well-informed choices about the integration of acupuncture into your treatment regimen.

Mindfulness Practices for Lung Health

Mindfulness practices can significantly improve lung health, complimenting medical treatments by promoting relaxation, reducing stress and improving breathing patterns.

Deep breathing exercises, such as diaphragmatic breathing, guided meditation and body scan meditation, can improve lung capacity and oxygen exchange.

Yoga practices like pranayama, which emphasise breath control, can enhance lung function and balance the respiratory system.

Gentle movement practices like Tai Chi or Qigong can improve fitness and lung capacity. Mindful stress reduction techniques, such as mindfulness-based stress reduction (MBSR), can help manage chronic stress.

Outdoor breathing exercises in nature can promote mindfulness, while conscious eating habits and positive self-talk can contribute to a healthier lifestyle. Conscious eating habits, such as chewing food slowly and savouring each bite, are essential for overall health.

Overall, mindfulness practices can contribute to overall well-being and lung health.

PART 7: Coping Strategies and Emotional Well-being

Dealing with Anxiety and Depression

Dealing with bronchitis can be challenging, and it's not uncommon for individuals to experience anxiety and depression during the recovery process.

To manage anxiety and depression during recovery from bronchitis, it is essential to consult with your medical expert, adhere to prescribed medications, engage in self-care practices, carry out deep breathing exercises, stay connected with friends and family and explore mindfulness and relaxation techniques.

Establish realistic goals for recovery and seek professional help if necessary. Maintain a healthy lifestyle by eating nutritious meals and staying hydrated.

Identify and minimise stressors in your life, such as scaling back on responsibilities or delegating tasks to others.

Physical and mental well-being are interconnected and addressing mental health concerns can contribute to a more holistic recovery. Engaging in self-care activities, such as warm baths, gentle exercise and adequate sleep, can help improve lung function and reduce anxiety.

Building a Support System

Having a strong support network is essential for managing bronchitis, since it may be a difficult and sometimes protracted respiratory ailment. *These techniques will assist you in creating a solid support network:*

Friends and Family:
Tell your close friends and relatives about your health. Tell them about your bronchitis, its symptoms and any special requirements you may have.

Ask close family members for emotional assistance. Having a confidante may sometimes have a big impact on how well you manage stress and anxiety.

Inform Your Circle of Support:
Make sure the people in your support network are aware of how bronchitis affects your day-to-day activities.

Provide accurate details on the illness, the recommended course of therapy and any possible side effects.

Inform them of the significance of avoiding contact with respiratory illnesses in order to keep your symptoms from becoming worse.

Honest Communication:
Maintain open channels of contact with your network of support. Talk about your emotions, worry and any modifications to your health.

Ensure that they are at ease enough to voice their concerns or ask inquiries.

Helpful Advice:

When experiencing a flare-up of bronchitis, ask for assistance with everyday duties like cooking, food shopping and housework.

Getting help with these duties may reduce your stress and free up your time so you can concentrate on getting well.

Complementary Healthcare Visits:
Ask a friend or member of your family to go with you to your doctor's visits. They may provide emotional support, ask questions and assist with taking notes.

It might also benefit to have someone with you to help you comprehend the treatment plan and suggestions made by the doctor.

Participate in Support Groups: Seek out support groups for people with respiratory issues, either locally or virtually. Making connections with others who are going through comparable struggles may be reassuring and insightful.

Social media groups and online forums may also be great places to exchange insights and guidance.

Support for Carers:

Make sure your caregiver has access to resources and assistance if you have one.

Giving advice and support may be advantageous for both parties, since caring for an individual with bronchitis can be taxing.

Emergency Procedure:

Talk to your support system about what to do in the event that your symptoms become worse.

Make sure they know your medical history, emergency contacts and any drugs you use.

Well-being and Self-Care:
Encourage the people in your support system to look for themselves. People who are caring for someone with bronchitis must put their own health first since it may be emotionally and physically taxing.

Living Positively with Bronchitis and Celebrating Small Victories

It might be difficult to live a happy life while you have bronchitis, but in order to manage the illness, you must concentrate on your little accomplishments and cultivate an optimistic outlook.

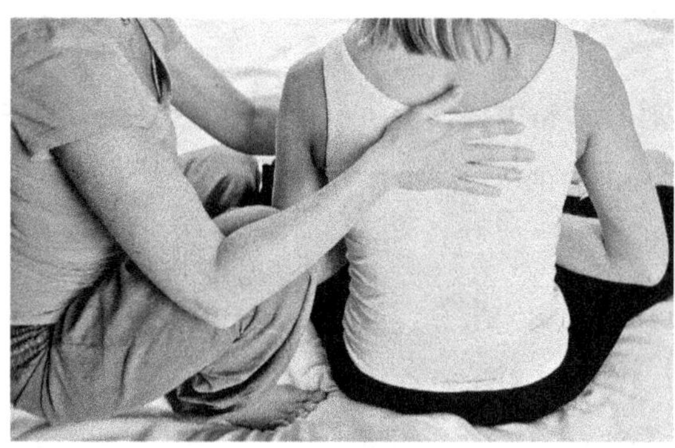

The following advice can help you manage your bronchitis and recognise your little victories along the way:

Recognise Your Limitations:

Acknowledge your physical limits and pay attention to your
health.

Recognise that you may sometimes need to prioritise rest and
self-care.

Set sensible objectives:

Establish attainable weekly or daily objectives that are in line
with your present state of health.
Celebrate even the littlest victories, like completing a home
chore or a quick workout.

Put Self-Care First:

Rest well so that your body can repair itself.

Consume enough amounts of water and relaxing drinks to stay
hydrated.

Adhere to your physician's advice and take prescription drugs
as recommended.

Perform Breathing Techniques:

Practise deep breathing techniques to alleviate stress and enhance lung function.

Breathing deeply and slowly might help calm you and clear your sinuses.

Remain Upbeat and Positive:

Instead of concentrating on the difficulties in your life, pay attention to the good things in it.
Be in the company of understanding and encouraging friends and relatives who are aware of your situation.

Celebrate Minor Victories:

Whether it's getting out of bed, taking a little walk or doing a home duty, acknowledge and appreciate every tiny win.

To track your achievements and development, keep a diary.

Sustain a Healthy Way of Life:

Maintain a balanced diet to boost your immune system and general well-being.

Light, low-impact exercise should be done as soon as your health permits.

Align Your Activities with Your Health:

Adapt your everyday routine to meet your health demands.

Seek for substitute activities that won't put too much pressure on your respiratory system for hobbies and socialising.

Seek Assistance and Support:

Join online forums or support groups to meet others going through similar experiences.

Talk about your experiences and take advice from those who have managed to live with bronchitis.

Acknowledge Advancement:

Think back on your trip and celebrate any accomplishments, no matter how little.

Make the most of setbacks as chances to grow and modify your strategy for improved health management.

Having bronchitis needs resilience and patience. To raise the quality of your life overall, acknowledge and appreciate the little things in life, put your health first and have an optimistic attitude.

PART 8: The Future of Bronchitis Management

Future Emerging Solutions and Research On Bronchitis

Treatment for chronic bronchitis is challenging as the illness progresses over time. Patients continue to have severe symptoms in spite of great efforts.

Many novel bronchoscopic therapies for this illness are currently being researched. Using various techniques, balloon desobstruction, bronchial rheoplasty and liquid nitrogen metered cryospray seek to eliminate the extra submucosal glands and hyperplastic goblet cells.

Clinical research on these medicines is still in its early stages, and bigger randomised controlled studies are required to validate the pilot data that is now available and assess the treatment's durability. Targeted lung denervation (TLD), the fourth procedure, involves ablating the parasympathetic nerves that run alongside the primary bronchi in an attempt to reduce the release of acetylcholine, which controls mucus production and smooth muscle tone.

Promising effects on the frequency of exacerbations have been shown and the evaluation of this medication is at a more advanced level. Confirmation of the improvement in symptoms related to chronic bronchitis is still required.

All of these therapies effectively target the emphysematous phenotype of COPD; nevertheless, their introduction has added to the body of information required to create novel bronchoscopic strategies for the chronic bronchitis phenotype.

In order to treat chronic bronchitis, we examine the most recent advancements in bronchoscopic surgery and analyse the relevant literature in this article.

For chronic bronchitis, there are currently three treatment options:

Stopping smoking, physical therapy ***(such as high-frequency chest wall oscillation, flutter valve, and chest physical therapy)*** and medication therapy ***(which includes mucolytics, expectorants, methylxanthines and short- and long-acting β-adrenergic receptor agonists, anticholinergics, glucocorticoids, phosphodiesterase (PDE)-4 inhibitors, antioxidants, and macrolides)***.

Nevertheless, despite great effort, patients still have severe symptoms since there are presently no authorised treatments that successfully address the airway metaplasia and mucus hypersecretion of chronic bronchitis. Alternative approaches to therapy are required.

The Role of Patient Advocacy

In order to properly treat bronchitis, patient advocacy is essential. An infection, either bacterial or viral, may induce bronchitis, which is an inflammation of the bronchial passages.

Here are some advantages of patient advocacy:

Patient Empowerment: Patients who actively participate in their healthcare are empowered by advocacy. It assists patients in comprehending their illness, available treatments and methods for self-care. Patients with bronchitis should understand how to treat their symptoms, when to get help and how to avoid complications.

Information Accessibility: Organisations and advocacy groups provide helpful bronchitis resources and information. This offers access to specialists, support groups, internet forums and instructional resources. Through advocacy channels, patients may find out about the most recent research, treatment recommendations and coping mechanisms.

Support Networks: For those suffering with bronchitis, patient advocacy fosters a caring environment. Patients may establish connections with others who are experiencing similar circumstances, exchange advice and provide emotional support.

Patients may feel less alone and be able to manage their illness more effectively with the support of this sense of community.

Increasing Awareness: Campaigns to avoid bronchitis and its symptoms, risk factors and treatments aim to increase public knowledge of these topics. This aids in raising awareness of the value of early identification, appropriate treatment and preventative actions among the general public, healthcare professionals, legislators and the media.

Promoting Healthcare Needs: Patient advocates strive to guarantee that people suffering with bronchitis have access to excellent medical treatment. This might include promoting more money for research, better treatment alternatives, more advanced diagnostic technologies and laws that protect patients' rights.

Encouraging Prevention: In order to lessen the incidence of bronchitis, advocacy activities are concentrated on encouraging preventative practices. This entails pushing for immunisation against pneumonia and the flu, encouraging hygienic breathing techniques and increasing knowledge of the environmental variables that might aggravate the symptoms of bronchitis.

Enhancing Care Coordination: For those who have bronchitis, patient advocacy may aid in bettering care coordination. In order to guarantee that patients get prompt and appropriate treatment, including access to specialists, prescription drugs and supporting services, advocates may collaborate with healthcare providers, insurers and other stakeholders.

In All, patient advocacy—which includes information, resources, support and lobbying for healthcare needs—plays a critical role in helping people with bronchitis. Advocacy initiatives improve results and quality of life for bronchitis patients by educating the public and empowering patients.

CONCLUSION

Looking Towards a Healthier You and a Brighter Future

It might be difficult to recover from bronchitis, but you can create the foundation for a better and healthier future with perseverance, the correct treatment and good habits.

These actions may help you heal and enhance your general wellbeing:

Rest and Relaxation:

Make sure you get enough sleep to give your body the time it needs to repair. For your immune system to properly fend off infections and expedite healing, you need to get enough sleep and relax.

Keep Yourself Hydrated:

To help calm your throat, thin mucus and keep your body hydrated, drink plenty of water, herbal teas and clear broths.

Steer clear of alcohol and caffeinated drinks since these might cause dehydration.

Observe Doctor's Orders:

If a medical practitioner diagnosed you with bronchitis, be sure to adhere to their recommended course of treatment. This might include taking drugs like bronchodilators, cough suppressants or antibiotics *(in the event that the bronchitis is bacterial)*.

Warm Compresses and Humidifiers:

To improve breathing comfort, use warm compresses to your chest or run a humidifier in your room to reduce chest congestion and soothe inflamed airways.

Avoid Irritants:

Steer clear of anything that might aggravate respiratory symptoms and lengthen healing time, such as air pollution, cigarette smoke, strong chemical smells and other irritants.

Mild Exercise:

Although relaxation is necessary, mild exercise like yoga, walking or stretching may aid with circulation, lung function and mood enhancement. Nevertheless, pay attention to your body and hold off on intense activity until you've completely healed.
Healthy Diet:

To boost your immune system and speed up healing, fill your body with wholesome meals high in vitamins, minerals and antioxidants. Make sure your diet is rich in whole grains, lean meats, fruits, veggies and healthy fats.

Maintain Good Hygiene:

To stop the transmission of germs, wash your hands often with soap and water. When you cough or sneeze, cover your mouth and nose with a tissue or your elbow to prevent spreading the infection to other people.

Keep an eye on your Symptoms:

Maintain a record of your symptoms and any changes to your health. See your doctor right away if your symptoms become worse or if you encounter any new issues.

Gradual Return to Normal Activities:

When you begin to feel better, go back to your regular activities little by bit, taking care not to push yourself too much. Give your body the time it needs to heal completely.

Do know that each person's road to recovery is different, so practise self-compassion and give your body the time and attention it needs. You may look forward to a better future free from bronchitis by being proactive in supporting your health and well-being.

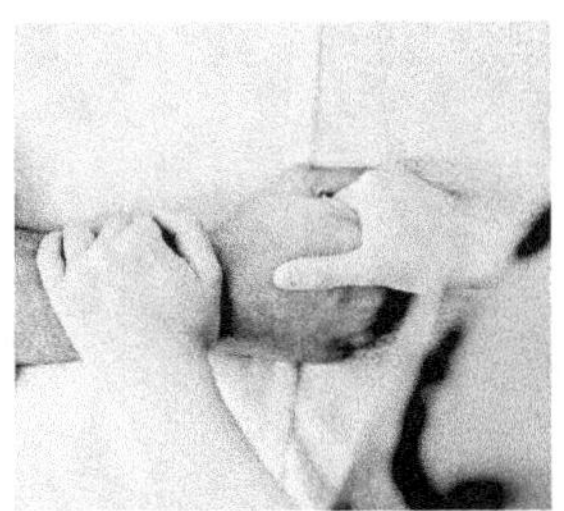

Get Well Soon ✿